# The Ultimate Anti Inflammatory Diet for Beginners

## Quick and Easy Anti-Inflammatory Recipes with 21 Day Meal Plan to Heal Your Immune System

# Table of Contents

# Introduction

Inflammation is a course correction measure used by the human body when it suffers an injury through pathogens, bacteria, a virus, or any harmful stimuli. The protective measure, which includes immune cells, blood vessels, and white blood cells, ensures that the aggravated body part gets help in repairing the damaged cell, making healing possible.

However, in certain cases, our immune system itself causes inflammation, even when there are no external stimuli to fight, such as in the case of arthritis. In this case, the autoimmune system treats the disease as a regular tissue disintegration, resulting in pain and inflammation.

While there are various ways to deal with inflammation, one of the most common and prescribed methods is to add food items with anti-inflammatory benefits to your diet. Research has shown that anti-inflammatory diet food is much more effective than medicines. When combined with a healthy lifestyle involving regular exercise, an anti-inflammatory diet has proven to be a boon not only for people from regular walks of life but also for athletes in whom wear and tear of muscles and body cells is a common phenomenon.

Keeping in mind the complexity of the program, here is a special guide that will help you understand inflammation in ways that no one else has been able to achieve so far. The aim behind this anti-inflammatory diet book is to not merely to provide you with recipes but also to make the process more spontaneous.

With abundant information available online and offline, it becomes very easy for the reader to get confused and lose interest. This adds to the pain that inflammation has caused already.

With the help of this book, you will understand everything about inflammation in a calculated manner that will be easy to grasp and implement. The book focuses on educating the reader through simple language, rather than waste energy proving the scientific prowess of the author.

The recipes mentioned in the book are easy to follow and involve ingredients that are readily available and have anti-inflammation properties.

By the time the reader begins to prepare their meals, the book will have educated them plenty about the best practices to counter the pain caused by inflammation. Along with the guidelines and tips to follow, the book contains a 21-day meal plan that will help you prepare a routine at your convenience.

The no-nonsense approach to the book helps us clear away the chatter and myths around inflammation, and helps you ease the pain that has been bothering you for so long.

# What Is Inflammation?

Inflammation is an autoimmune tactic developed by the human body to fight back against a certain disease, infection, or injury. We all undergo inflammation; sometimes, it's visible outside the body, and other times it's not. When the body meets certain conditions, inflammation can result. Inflammation is an order of our immune system's defense mechanism to keep us safe. If it weren't for inflammation, many injuries would take longer to heal or would not heal at all.

Inflammation happens as a response of the body tissues when we get in contact with a harmful stimulant which may include an attack by pathogens, damaged cells due to injury, or irritants of any other nature.

Inflammation is carried out with the help of actions by our immune cells, along with the blood vessels, and molecular mediators such as inflammatory cytokines. Inflammation is the first line of defense in the human body as it prevents the harmful pathogen from aggravating the disease or pain to the body. It also affirms that the initial blow to the body leads to minimizing cell damage and helps in clearing necrotic cells from the spot of the attack. This assists in helping the body to initiate a speedy tissue repair process. Some of the common indicators of inflammation are heat, swelling, redness, acute pain, and loss of function.

Inflammation can be classified into two groups: acute or chronic inflammation. Acute inflammation is a condition that develops due to the body's response to an outside attack. This inflammation is a result of the increase in the plasma and leukocyte movement in the body. During this process, the granulocytes, a special kind of white blood cell with granules, are flown into the injured tissues through the blood. This catalyzes the biochemical event that helps to soothe the attacked area and results in the inflammatory response of the human body. Acute inflammation is the first response shown by the human body to any outer grievances. This acts immediately upon the injury and lasts for only a few days before being completely healed. Cytokines and chemokines in the body facilitate the neutrophils and macrophages to move to the inflamed area to heal it. Any inflammation that lasts six weeks is categorized as acute inflammation.

On the other hand, in the case of chronic inflammation, the body undergoes pain and inflammation that can last for months or even years. Unlike with acute inflammation, in which neutrophils take charge, in chronic inflammation, they are replaced by macrophages, plasma cells, and lymphocytes. Some common examples of such cases are diabetes, cardiovascular ailments, allergies, and pulmonary disease. Some of the prime reasons attached to chronic inflammation are obesity, poor eating habits, smoking, and stress.

Inflammation is one of the most common injuries faced by athletes and anyone on a physical workout regime. This usually happens when the human body undergoes grinding. The body is self-sufficient in recovering from inflammation. However, one should not undermine and overlook when the pain and inflammation is sustained for a longer period. From various food items to exercise, there are different ways that a person can treat inflammation with ease. Various causes can lead to inflammation in the body. One of the common factors is irritants or foreign materials that the human body is not able to process easily. One should also be mindful if the body starts showing signs of recurrent episodes of inflammation. If not treated on time, the inflammation can also result in chronic disorder. Foods such as processed sugar, refined carbs, alcohol, processed meat, and fats have shown the property of increasing the chances of causing or worsening inflammation in people.

# Common Symptoms of Inflammation

Inflammation is one of the most common issues faced by the human body. Be it someone engaged in harsh physical activity like athletes or any health enthusiasts, anyone can be caught by inflammation. Though inflammation is the human body's response to an irritant (the irritant, in this case, could be a germ inside the body or a foreign particle), any inflammation should not be ignored. When the body part gets hurt, the wound swells up, turns red, and causes pain. This is a common sign of inflammation. Therefore, the inflammation not only will be initiated when the body suffers an outer blow but can be a result of the body having been attacked by the germ, leading the body to not being able to heal properly.

Some of the most common agents of inflammation are:

**Pathogens**: These are organisms such as bacteria, fungi, or viruses that will result in the formation of the disease. It should be noted that the human body already contains microbes that can cause the problem to our immune systems. When left untreated for a long time, the microbes start to fight and weaken the immune system. However, the pathogens can cause dysfunction of the immune system upon entering the body externally.

**External injuries**: When the body suffers a blow from the outside, it may result in external injury. In this case, if the wound is left unattended or not treated on time, it may lead the affected party to show signs of inflammation. Getting a scrape on any body part that can lead to redness and accumulation of pus is a type of external injury that will result in some form of inflammation.

Chemical injury: At times when the body is exposed to harsh chemicals, it will lead to redness and swelling in the skin.

**Medical conditions**: Various medical conditions upon the absence of treatment can also aggravate the inflammation inside the body, resulting in low immunity and pain. Some of the inflammation-causing diseases are cystitis (inflammation of the bladder); bronchitis (inflammation in bronchi); otitis media (inflammation in the middle ear); or dermatitis (inflammation of the skin).

Of all types of inflammation, the injuries have some common traits that can help a person identify the disease. Some of the common symptoms that are signs of acute inflammation in a person are:

Redness: This is one of the most common symptoms of inflammation. Whenever a person is attacked by an external agent, it causes the place of impact to turn red. This redness can easily be identified by the naked eye. However, in certain cases, doctors will require the expertise of dedicated equipment if the impact of the injury is inside the human body.

**Heat**: At times when the body part takes a blow or gets infected by a pathogen, the affected body part will show signs of heat. In some cases, the body may also develop fever and raise the temperature. This is another symptom of inflammation.

**Swelling**: This is the most common and easily identified symptom of inflammation. As the autoimmune system of the body starts treating the injury, it results in swelling in a particular area.

**Pain**: Inflammation in certain cases can also lead to acute pain in the human body or the aggravated area. The level of pain denotes the severity of the blow or injury. The pain can arise due to the outer impact or can be internal as well. It is advised that the person should not treat pain lightly and should consult a medic if the problem persists.

**Loss of function**: In certain cases when the injury is chronic, it may also result in the person losing vital functions. This might mean that the patient's body is also suffering from inflammation. Some of the most common examples include loss of movement due to pain or inflammation in the joints. Difficulty breathing is another symptom that may be due to inflammation.

Other than these, flu-like symptoms can also be a reminder of inflammation. Some of the most common are fever, chills, cough, shortness of breath, cold, fatigue, headache, loss of energy, appetite loss, and stiffness in the muscle.

Inflammation does not necessarily follow the mentioned symptoms. In some cases, inflammation may be an internal factor and not known to the person. Therefore, a doctor should be consulted if the person is not at ease. Some known inflammations have proved to show zero symptoms until diagnosed by a professional.

# Health Risks of Inflammation

Though inflammation is a very common factor in the human body, when the inflammation does not subside within a short period and is left untreated, it can lead to various complications in the smooth functioning of the body.

Inflammation generally means that the human immune system is busy responding to a threat or an injury that the person may have received. As the injured area becomes red due to the impact, the white blood cells flow toward it to heal it as fast as possible. The body reacts similarly in the case of an internal injury. This is the general course of action for the body. However, there may be instances when the human body is not able to take care of the inflammation on its own or is taking a long time to heal. This happens if the human body lacks immunity or does not have enough white blood cells to fight back due to deficiency in the body. In another case, it might be possible that due to the size and complexity of the injury, the healing of inflammation takes longer than usual. This is when the person should seek help from an expert and not let the problem persist any further.

It is also observed that in certain cases, the inflammation does not work in its orderly fashion. Here, the immune response of inflammation occurs even when the body did not suffer any breakdown or external injury. Therefore, the body of the person develops inflammation, but the immune system does not heal it for long, causing pain and other disorders in the human body.

Some of the common examples of such events occur if the person is suffering from obesity, stress, or other autoimmune disorders. This kind of abnormal inflammation is identified as the chronic state of inflammation.

When left unattended, risks due to inflammation can lead to various health problems in a person. Some of the most common ones are heart ailments, arthritis, depression, cancer, and Alzheimer's disease.

While acute inflammation has been shown to subside over a short period, it is chronic inflammation that leads to various disorders and affects the healthy living of a person. Over a while, chronic inflammation can also initiate the reverse immune system response. This is when the immune system of the body, instead of protecting, starts to attack the healthy tissues and healthy body organs. Diabetes, cancer, and rheumatoid arthritis are some of the most common causes of unlawful inflammation.

To combat inflammation, the person should immediately consult a doctor and get diagnosed. Once the problem is identified, the doctor will help the person with medicines and certain measures to ensure that the inflammation does not spread and disturb immunity.

One of the primary methods of challenging inflammation is by following a healthy lifestyle that includes exercise and a well-balanced diet. This is arguably the best approach to defeating the ailments that accompany inflammation. The person should avoid food items that can cause or aggravate chronic inflammation. Red meat, processed carbs, deep-fried foods, and processed sugar should be avoided at all costs. Opting to go for all green vegetables, seasonal fruits, nuts, fish, and olive oil can greatly treat the concern of inflammation. Also, it is advised that the person should be involved in a daily exercise routine while maintaining a healthy sleep pattern. Most importantly, keeping the mind away from stress works wonders in such cases.

# Guidelines for the Anti-Inflammatory Diet

It has been long proven that to combat inflammation, a person should focus more on their kitchen rather than paying doctors' bills. While a doctor is very necessary if the person develops chronic inflammation, no one can counter the benefits of a healthy meal, which is one of the main prescriptions given by doctors as well.

Though not very specific, an anti-inflammatory diet focuses on replacing all food items like processed carbs, deep-fried foods, red meat, alcohol, and processed sugar with foods such as fruits and green leafy vegetables, fatty, omega-3 fatty acids, whole grains, lean protein, and spices.

While there are no certain guidelines to adopt a particular anti-inflammatory diet, the basic guideline argues against using certain foods that have shown a tendency to aggravate or even catalyze inflammation. Dairy products, processed foods, foods with added sugar or salt, unhealthy oils, processed carbs, baked goods, processed snacks, nightshades, legumes, eggs, premade desserts, alcohol including wine, refined carbohydrates, fried foods, soda, carbonated sugar beverages, red meat, steaks, processed meat, and margarine have all been shown to have adverse effects for anyone suffering from inflammation.

While deciding to go for an anti-inflammatory diet, the person should be more focused on selecting all-natural food items, and good sources of antioxidants. A well-balanced anti-inflammatory diet will always include foods that are rich in antioxidants and limit the production of free radicals in the human body. Some research has also shown that a careful selection between a Mediterranean diet and the DASH diet that involves fresh fruits, green leafy vegetables, and fish is a good start to an anti-inflammatory diet.

Besides this, some general guidelines that will go a long way in ensuring a good anti-inflammatory meal are:

**A mix of diets:** Always remember that there is no one food item or method to maintain good health, or to fight inflammation in this case. The person should look for all the practical options available and then choose a variety of healthy ingredients before deciding on the meal. To consume an anti-inflammatory diet, the body should not be deprived of other necessary nutrients it requires for proper functioning.

**Fresh is the key:** Whenever you have to purchase food items, remember to go for fresh foods. Food on shelves for long periods loses its nutritional value and thus will not be as effective as it should. Even when you want to prepare your meal in advance, one should look for food items that will not lose their value until consumed. There is very little difference between eating processed foods and food that has lost its freshness.

**Check the information on labels:** One of the most important tasks before purchasing food is to check the entire ingredient list or the nutritional value of the packet. Premade foods such as cocoa at times contain processed sugar and fat and should be avoided.

**Consume good-looking food:** There is nothing as good as a plate filled with various food items. Remember that to cure inflammation does not mean that you cannot enjoy eating. Choose food items that you like and that will attract you.

# Tips for the Anti-Inflammatory Diet

Just like any change, getting used to an anti-inflammatory diet can be a bit difficult for beginners. However, the change in diet is not a significant alteration from what we eat anyway; it's the discipline that tends to particularly lead people to give up halfway into the process.

Some of the tips that will be helpful to make the transition a happy phase are:

**Choose what you love:** Given the various food items that one can consume while on an anti-inflammatory diet, the person should begin by choosing recipes containing the foods that they particularly like to eat. Only once you start enjoying your meals and are also able to keep a disciplined schedule, start adding other food items to the menu to get a wholesome experience.

**Pick a variety of foods:** It is often said that good-looking food evokes the senses and helps us enjoy the meal much more than eating similar foods that might become challenging and mundane to consume. Therefore, whenever you decide to fill your grocery cart, include fruits and vegetables that are not only fresh but also colorful.

**Change is a slow process:** When one decides to start with an anti-inflammatory diet, it is advised to not jump into the plan with all guns blazing. Remember that your body needs time to adapt to new dieting habits. Therefore, the person should gradually take small steps before starting a full-fledged diet. The same applies in the case of snacks. We all love too many snacks and therefore should replace unhealthy snacks with salads filled with crunchy green vegetables.

Likewise, one should replace processed fast-food meals with homemade foods and soda with mineral water.

Another important tip to keep in mind is to visit your doctor regularly. You should decide on the intensity of your anti-inflammatory meal only after consulting the doctor if you are suffering from chronic inflammation. Any use of supplements or multivitamins should also be brought to the attention of the doctor looking after your medical condition.

Being involved in a healthy lifestyle with daily moderate exercise and getting proper sleep also adds to the benefits you will achieve through an anti-inflammatory diet.

# Food to Eat and Avoid on the Anti-Inflammatory Diet

Any all-natural food item, including seasonal fruits, green vegetables, whole grains, plant proteins, fatty fish, herbs, and spices, all show anti-inflammation properties.

**Foods to Eat on the Anti-Inflammatory Diet:**

Colorful and seasonal fruits

Green leafy vegetables

Broccoli

Kale

Spinach

Cabbage

Oatmeal

Brown rice

Whole-wheat bread

Unrefined grains with fiber

Beans

Nuts

Fish

Herbs

Spices

Turmeric

Curcumin

Contrary to that, anything that is heavily processed, carbonated sugar drinks, oily food, fried food items, and alcohol are major causes of inflammation.

**Food to Avoid on the Anti-Inflammatory Diet:**

Processed foods

Foods with added sugar or salt

Unhealthy oils

Processed carbs

White bread, white pasta

Baked goods, cookies

Processed snack foods, such as chips, crackers, and fries

Nightshades

Legumes

Eggs

Premade desserts, ice cream

Alcohol including wine

Refined carbohydrates

Fried foods

Soda

Sugar-sweetened beverages

Red meat

Processed meat

Margarine

# 21-Day Meal Plan

| Day | Breakfast | Lunch | Dinner |
|---|---|---|---|
| 1 | Cherry Mocha Breakfast Smoothie | Ground Turkey Bowl | Creamy Broccoli Soup + Roasted Broccoli with Potatoes |
| 2 | Kale and Avocado Omelet | Herbed Cod with Capers and Roasted Tomatoes | Ground Turkey Bowl |
| 3 | Lemon-Pistachio Labneh | Scallops Served with White Beans | Grilled Corn and Veggie Salad |
| 4 | Berries and Mascarpone Toast | Chicken, Kale, and Lemon Orzo Soup | Mustard Flavored Salmon + Garlic Kale |
| 5 | Peanut Butter and Jelly Smoothie | Arugula and Citrus Pork Salad | Grilled Chicken with Cauliflower Rice |
| 6 | Baked Walnut, Raisin and Banana Oatmeal | Chicken and Veggies with Lemon Couscous | Roasted Cauliflower |
| 7 | Whole-Wheat Orange Pancakes | Minestrone Vegan Soup + Roasted Broccoli with Potatoes | Grilled Chicken with Cauliflower Rice |
| 8 | Spinach and Smoked Trout Scrambled Eggs | Saag Paneer | Chicken and Veggies with Lemon Couscous |
| 9 | Baked Walnut, Raisin and Banana Oatmeal | Teriyaki Turkey Delight + Grilled Peppers | Massaman Chicken Curry with Turmeric Rice |

| | | | |
|---|---|---|---|
| 10 | Whole-Wheat Orange Pancakes | Ginger and Mango Barbequed Chicken | Vegan Cauliflower Salad |
| 11 | Cherry Mocha Breakfast Smoothie | Spicy Eggplant Bhartha | Garlic-Flavored Roasted Salmon and Brussels Sprouts |
| 12 | Kale and Avocado Omelet | Crusted Mustard Potatoes + Grilled Citrus Asparagus | Massaman Chicken Curry with Turmeric Rice |
| 13 | Lemon-Pistachio Labneh | Curried Peanut and Sweet Potato Soup | Potato and Chickpea Curry |
| 14 | Spinach and Smoked Trout Scrambled Eggs | Spicy Chicken and Quinoa Bowl + Coleslaw (Sweet and Sour) | Quick and Easy Shrimp Scampi + Roasted Broccoli with Potatoes |
| 15 | Peanut Butter and Jelly Smoothie | Tilapia Fillets Served with Pecans and Orange | Chicken Tikka Masala |
| 16 | Whole-Wheat Orange Pancakes | Spicy Chicken and Quinoa Bowl | Rosemary and Walnut Crusted Salmon |
| 17 | Cherry Mocha Breakfast Smoothie | Fresh Avocado and Orange Salad + Roasted Turmeric Sweet Potatoes | Red Pepper Flavored Quinoa with Salmon + Coleslaw (Sweet and Sour) |
| 18 | Kale and Avocado Omelet | Kale and Bean Stuffed Sweet Potato | Mediterranean Chickpea and Chicken Soup |
| 19 | Lemon-Pistachio Labneh | Mediterranean Chickpea and Chicken Soup | Tilapia Fillets Served with Pecans and Orange |
| | | Mediterranean Fresh | |

| | | | |
|---|---|---|---|
| 20 | Berries and Mascarpone Toast | Lettuce Wraps + Italian-Style Spinach and Mushrooms | Watercress, Pear, and Roquefort Salad |
| 21 | Peanut Butter and Jelly Smoothie | Teriyaki Turkey Delight + Garlic Kale | Kale and Bean Stuffed Sweet Potato |

# Anti-Inflammatory Breakfast Recipes

## Cherry Mocha Breakfast Smoothie

**Serving Size: 1**
**Servings per Recipe: 2**
**Calories: 272 calories per serving**
**Total Time: 10 minutes**

**Ingredients:**

Frozen dark sweet cherries (unsweetened) – 1 cup

Chocolate almond milk (unsweetened) – 1 cup

Vanilla Greek yogurt (fat-free) – 5.3-ounce carton

Banana – ½ medium

Cocoa powder (unsweetened) – 2 tablespoons

Almond butter – 2 tablespoons

Coffee powder (instant espresso) – 1 teaspoon

Vanilla – 1 teaspoon

Ice cubes – 2 cups

Dark chocolate shavings – 1 tablespoon

Espresso beans (chocolate-covered) – 1 tablespoon

**Nutrition Information:**

Fat – 12 g

Protein – 13 g

Carbohydrates – 34 g

**Directions:**

1. Start by taking a blender and adding in the banana, cherries, Greek yogurt, almond milk, cocoa powder, espresso coffee powder,

vanilla, and almond butter.

2. Blend until all ingredients are well incorporated and form a smooth, puree-like consistency.

3. Add in the ice cubes and blend well.

4. Pour into 2 tall glasses and top each glass with ½ tablespoon of chocolate shavings and espresso beans.

5. Serve right away!


## Kale and Avocado Omelet

**Serving Size: 1**
**Servings per Recipe: 1**
**Calories: 339 calories per serving**
**Total Time: 10 minutes**

**Ingredients:**

Eggs – 2 large

Milk (2%) – 1 teaspoon

Salt – as required

Olive oil (extra-virgin) – 2 teaspoons

Kale (chopped) – 1 cup

Lime juice – 1 tablespoon

Fresh cilantro (chopped) – 1 tablespoon

Sunflower seeds – 1 teaspoon

Red pepper (crushed) – ⅛ teaspoon

Avocado (sliced) – ¼

**Nutrition Information:**

Fat – 28.1 g

Protein – 15 g

Carbohydrates – 8.6 g

## Directions:

1. Take a small bowl and add in the eggs, milk, and a pinch of salt. Beat until well combined.
2. Place a small nonstick skillet on a medium flame and pour 1 teaspoon of oil over the same.
3. Once the oil is hot enough, pour the egg and milk mixture; cook for a couple of minutes. Flip over and cook for another 30 seconds.
4. Transfer onto a plate and set aside.
5. Take a large mixing bowl and add in the kale, 1 teaspoon of oil, cilantro, lime juice, crushed red pepper, a pinch of salt, and sunflower seeds. Toss well until kale leaves are evenly coated.
6. Place the kale mixture over the omelet and finish by placing the slices on top.
7. Serve right away!

## Lemon-Pistachio Labneh

**Serving Size: ¼ cup**
**Servings per Recipe: 8**
**Calories: 108 calories per serving**
**Total Time: 12 hours**

## Ingredients:

Plain yogurt (low-fat) – 4 cups

Salt – ¼ teaspoon

Pistachios (shelled) – ¼ cup

Lemon oil – 1 tablespoon

Fresh parsley (chopped) – 1 tablespoon

Lemon zest – 1 teaspoon

Sumac (ground) – ¼ teaspoon

**Nutrition Information:**

Fat – 5.3 g

Protein – 7 g

Carbohydrates – 8.3 g

**Directions:**

1. Take a large mesh sieve and line it with 4 layers of cheesecloth. Place the sieve over a bowl and set aside.
2. Take a glass mixing bowl and add in the yogurt along with some salt. Whisk well until smooth. Transfer the mixture over the cheesecloth. Let it sit overnight to ensure all liquid is drained into the bowl below.
3. Once done, transfer the drained yogurt into a bowl and stir well.
4. Serve by topping the yogurt with oil, parsley, pistachios, sumac, and lemon zest.

## Berries and Mascarpone Toast

**Serving Size: 1**
**Servings per Recipe: 1**
**Calories: 326 calories per serving**
**Total Time: 7 minutes**

**Ingredients:**

Whole-grain bread – 1 slice

Mascarpone cheese – 2 tablespoons

Mixed berries – ¼ cup

Mint leaves – 1 teaspoon

## Nutrition Information:

Fat – 27.3 g

Protein – 7.9 g

Carbohydrates – 15.1 g

## Directions:

1. Begin by toasting the bread slice until golden brown.
2. Spread the mascarpone cheese evenly over the toasted slice.
3. Finish by topping the cheese on the toast with mixed berries and mint leaves.
4. Enjoy!

## Peanut Butter and Jelly Smoothie

**Serving Size: 1**
**Servings per Recipe: 1**
**Calories: 367 calories per serving**
**Total Time: 5 minutes**

## Ingredients:

Milk (skimmed) – ½ cup

Plain Greek yogurt (nonfat) – ⅓ cup

Baby spinach – 1 cup

Banana slices (frozen) – 1 cup

Strawberries (frozen) – ½ cup

Natural peanut butter – 1 tablespoon

Pure maple syrup – 1-2 teaspoons

## Nutrition Information:

Fat – 10.2 g

Protein – 18.1 g

Carbohydrates – 53.9 g

**Directions:**

1. Start by taking a blender and adding in the yogurt and milk.
2. Toss in the spinach, strawberries, banana, sweetener, and peanut butter; blend into a smooth, puree-like consistency.
3. Transfer into a tall glass and serve!

## Baked Walnut, Raisin, and Banana Oatmeal

**Serving Size: 1**
**Servings per Recipe: 6**
**Calories: 327 calories per serving**
**Total Time: 1 hour 5 minutes**

**Ingredients:**

Rolled oats – 2 cups

Walnuts (chopped) – ⅓ cup

Cinnamon (ground) – 1 ½ teaspoons

Baking powder – 1 teaspoon

Salt – ½ teaspoon

Allspice (ground) – ¼ teaspoon

Milk (skimmed) – 2 cups

Plain yogurt (low-fat) – ¾ cup

Canola oil – 2 tablespoons

Light brown sugar – ¼ cup

Vanilla extract – 1 teaspoon

Banana (halved and sliced) – 1 large

Raisins – ⅓ cup

**Nutrition Information:**

Fat – 13.1 g

Protein – 9.1 g

Carbohydrates – 46.2 g

**Directions:**

1. Begin by preheating the oven by setting the temperature to 375 degrees Fahrenheit.
2. Take a square glass baking dish and grease it generously with cooking spray.
3. In a large mixing bowl, add in the oats, cinnamon, walnuts, baking powder, allspice, and salt. Mix well to combine.
4. In another bowl, add in the yogurt, milk, oil, vanilla, and brown sugar; whisk well.
5. Transfer the yogurt and milk mixture into the oats mixture and combine until all ingredients are well incorporated.
6. Add in the raisins and bananas and fold them using a spatula. Pour the prepared batter into the prepared square dish.
7. Place the baking dish into the preheated oven and bake for about 45 minutes or until the top of the oatmeal is golden and firm.
8. Serve!

## Whole-Wheat Orange Pancakes

**Serving Size: 2**
**Servings per Recipe: 6**
**Calories: 248 calories per serving**
**Total Time: 30 minutes**

**Ingredients:**

Whole -wheat flour – 1 ½ cups

Flaxmeal – 3 tablespoons

Baking powder – 1 ½ teaspoons

Baking soda – ½ teaspoon

Ground ginger – ¼ teaspoon

Salt – ⅛ teaspoon

Oranges – 3

Buttermilk – 1 ¼ cups

Eggs – 2 large

Vanilla extract – 1 teaspoon

Brown sugar (packed) – 2 tablespoons

Canola oil – 2 tablespoons

**Nutrition Information:**

Fat – 9 g

Protein – 8.8 g

Carbohydrates – 35.5 g

**Directions:**

1. Start by taking a large mixing bowl and add in the flour, baking powder, flaxmeal, baking soda, salt, and ginger. Whisk to combine.
2. Use a zester to zest one of the oranges and set aside. Juice the orange (you will get about ¼ cup of juice) and set aside.
3. Peel the remaining oranges and cut the segments into 3 pieces each. Transfer into a bowl and set aside.
4. Take a medium-sized mixing bowl and add in the buttermilk, vanilla, eggs, brown sugar, orange zest, orange juice, and oil. Whisk well to combine.
5. Pour the prepared buttermilk mixture into the flour mixture and mix well. Let the batter sit at room temperature for around 5

minutes.

6. In the meantime, take a nonstick pan and place it on a medium-high flame. Coat the pan lightly with cooking spray.

7. Use a measuring cup to scoop out the ⅓ cup of batter and drop it on the pan. Cook for about 3 minutes. Flip over and cook for another 2 minutes. Transfer onto a serving platter. Repeat the process with the remaining batter.

8. Top the pancakes with the cut orange segments and serve!

## Spinach and Smoked Trout Scrambled Eggs

**Serving Size: 1**
**Servings per Recipe: 2**
**Calories: 243 calories per serving**
**Total Time: 15 minutes**

### Ingredients:

Eggs – 4 large

Milk (reduced-fat) – 2 tablespoons

Ground pepper – ¼ teaspoon

Salt – a pinch

Avocado oil – 2 teaspoons

Shallot (finely chopped) – 2 tablespoons

Smoked trout (boned and flaked) – ½ cup

Spinach (chopped) – 1 cup

### Nutrition Information:

Fat – 16.7 g

Protein – 19 g

Carbohydrates – 3.9 g

### Directions:

1. Start by whisking eggs, pepper, salt, and milk in a medium-sized mixing bowl. The color of the mixture should be pale yellow.
2. Take a medium-sized nonstick skillet and place it on a medium flame. Pour in the oil and let it heat through.
3. Once the oil is hot enough, add in the shallot and sauté for about a couple of minutes or until the shallots are slightly browned.
4. Add in the whisked egg mixture and give it a quick, gentle stir. Reduce the flame to medium-low immediately and let the eggs cook for about 30 seconds.
5. Sprinkle the flaked trout evenly over the eggs. Scramble the eggs and cook for about 4 minutes.
6. Toss in the spinach and stir well; cook for about a minute or until the spinach is wilted.
7. Transfer onto a serving platter and serve!

# Anti-Inflammatory Soups and Salads Recipes

## Chicken, Kale, and Lemon Orzo Soup

**Serving Size: 1 ½ cups**
**Servings per Recipe: 6**
**Calories: 245 calories per serving**
**Total Time: 40 minutes**

**Ingredients:**

   Olive oil (extra-virgin) – 2 tablespoons

   Chicken breasts (boneless and skinless) – 1 pound

   Dried oregano – 1 teaspoon

   Salt – 1 ¼ teaspoons

   Ground pepper – ¾ teaspoon

   Onions (chopped) – 2 cups

   Carrots (chopped) – 1 cup

   Celery (chopped) – 1 cup

   Garlic (minced) – 2 cloves

   Bay leaf – 1

   Chicken broth (unsalted) – 4 cups

   Orzo pasta (whole-wheat) – ⅔ cup

   Kale (chopped) – 4 cups

   Lemon (zest and juice) – 1

**Nutrition Information:**

   Fat – 7 g

   Protein – 21.1 g

Carbohydrates – 24.2 g

## Directions:

1. Begin by trimming the chicken breasts and cutting them into bite-sized pieces.

2. Place a large stockpot on a medium-high flame and pour in 1 tablespoon of oil. Once the oil is hot enough, toss in the chicken pieces and season them with pepper, salt, and oregano. Stir and cook for about 5 minutes or until the chicken is lightly browned on the edges.

3. Once done, transfer the chicken onto a plate and set aside.

4. Pour the remaining oil into the stockpot and let it heat through. Add in the chopped onions, celery, and carrots and sauté for around 5 minutes. The veggies should be lightly browned and tender.

5. Add in the bay leaf, garlic, and remaining oregano. Stir well and cook for about 30 seconds.

6. Pour the broth into the veggies and increase the flame to high. Let the broth come to a boil and reduce the flame to low; cook for about 5 minutes.

7. Toss in the chicken and kale; cook for about 8 minutes. The chicken should be thoroughly cooked by now.

8. Turn off the flame and add in the lemon juice, lemon zest, pepper, and salt. Stir until all ingredients are well incorporated.

9. Serve hot!

## Minestrone Vegan Soup

**Serving Size: 1**
**Servings per Recipe: 6**
**Calories: 267 calories per serving**
**Total Time: 30 minutes**

**Ingredients:**

    Garlic (minced) – 5 cloves

    Olive oil (extra-virgin) – 3 tablespoons

    Whole-grain bread (cubed) – 1 cup

    Leek (rinsed and chopped) – 1 cup

    Carrots (chopped) – 1 cup

    Vegetable broth (low-sodium) – 3 cups

    Water – 3 cups

    Kosher salt – ¾ teaspoon

    Ditalini pasta – 1 cup

    Zucchini (halved and sliced) – 1 medium

    Cannellini beans (no added salt) – 1 can (15 ounce)

    Baby kale (fresh) – 3 cups

    Frozen peas (thawed) – 1 cup

    Ground pepper – ½ teaspoon

**Nutrition Information:**

    Fat – 8.6 g

    Protein – 9.7 g

    Carbohydrates – 38.7 g

**Directions:**

1. Begin by preheating the oven by setting the temperature to 350 degrees Fahrenheit.
2. Place a medium-sized skillet on a medium flame and pour in 2 tablespoons of oil.
3. Once the oil is heated, add in the garlic and cook for about 4 minutes, stirring continuously.

4. Toss in the cubed bread and stir until evenly coated. Transfer the sautéed bread cubes onto a baking sheet and bake for around 8-10 minutes.

5. In the meantime, place a large stockpot on a medium-high flame. Pour 1 tablespoon of oil into the same.

6. Once the oil is hot enough, add in the chopped carrots and leek; stir and cook for around 5 minutes.

7. Pour in the water and broth along with the salt. Increase the flame to high and let it come to a boil.

8. Once the water and broth mixture boils, toss in the pasta and stir. Reduce the flame to medium-high and cook for about 5 minutes.

9. Toss in the thinly sliced zucchini and cook for another 5 minutes. Keep stirring to prevent the pasta from sticking to the bottom.

10. Now add in the beans, pepper, and kale; cook for another 2 minutes or until kale is wilted.

11. Transfer the prepared soup into a bowl and top with croutons.

12. Serve hot!

## Curried Peanut and Sweet Potato Soup

**Serving Size: 1**
**Servings per Recipe: 6**
**Calories: 345 calories per serving**
**Total Time: 40 minutes**

**Ingredients:**

Canola oil – 2 tablespoons

Yellow onion (diced) – 1 ½ cups

Garlic (minced) – 1 tablespoon

Fresh ginger (minced) – 1 tablespoon

Red curry paste – 4 teaspoons

Serrano chile (seeds removed and minced) – 1

Sweet potato (peeled and cubed) – 1 pound

Water – 3 cups

Coconut milk (lite) – 1 cup

Dry-roasted peanuts (unsalted) – ¾ cup

White beans (rinsed) – 1 can (15 ounce)

Salt – ¾ teaspoon

Pepper (freshly ground) – ¼ teaspoon

Fresh cilantro (chopped) – ¼ cup

Lime juice – 2 tablespoons

Roasted pumpkin seeds (unsalted) –

¼ cup Lime wedges

## Nutrition Information:

Fat – 19.4 g

Protein – 12.6 g

Carbohydrates – 37.4 g

## Directions:

1. Start by cutting the sweet potatoes into ½-inch cubes. Transfer them into a bowl and set aside.
2. Take a large pot and place it on a medium-high flame. Pour in the oil and let it heat through.
3. Add in the onion and sauté for around 4 minutes. Also add in the ginger, garlic, Serrano, and curry paste and sauté for another 1 minute.
4. Now add in the cubed sweet potatoes and cook on a medium-low flame for about 12 minutes or until the potatoes become tender.

5. Take a blender and transfer about half of the soup into the same. Also, add in the peanuts and coconut milk. Blend into a smooth, puree-like consistency.

6. Return the pureed soup to the stockpot and mix well.

7. Add in the beans, pepper, and salt; stir well and let it heat through. Remove from the flame and add in the lime juice and chopped cilantro.

8. Transfer into a serving bowl and top with lime wedges and pumpkin seeds.

9. Serve hot!

## Creamy Broccoli Soup

**Serving Size: 1**
**Servings per Recipe: 6**
**Calories: 157 calories per serving**
**Total Time: 30 minutes**

**Ingredients:**

Butter (unsalted) – 3 tablespoons

Leeks (rinsed and sliced) – 2 medium

Celery (thinly sliced) – ½ cup

Garlic (finely chopped) – 1 clove

Broccoli florets – 8 cups

Vegetable broth (low-sodium) – 4 cups

Fresh thyme leaves – 1 teaspoon

Salt – ½ teaspoon

Half-and-half – 1 cup

Chives (thinly sliced) – 2 teaspoons

**Nutrition Information:**

Fat – 10.4 g

Protein – 4.7 g

Carbohydrates – 13.4 g

## Directions:

1. Begin by placing a large nonstick saucepan on a medium-high flame. Add in the butter and let them melt through.
2. Toss in the chopped celery and leeks; cook for about 8 minutes. Keep stirring to prevent the veggies from sticking to the bottom.
3. Add in the garlic and stir for about a minute until fragrant.
4. Now add in the broth and broccoli florets and let it come to a boil. Reduce the flame to medium and cook for around 12 minutes until the broccoli becomes tender.
5. Sprinkle with salt and thyme; stir well. Remove from the flame.
6. Use an immersion blender to puree the broccoli and broth into a smooth, puree-like consistency.
7. Add in the half-and-half and blend again until all ingredients are well incorporated.
8. Transfer into a serving bowl and garnish with chives.
9. Serve right away!

## Mediterranean Chickpea and Chicken Soup

**Serving Size: 1**
**Servings per Recipe: 6**
**Calories: 447 calories per serving**
**Total Time: 1 hour 20 minutes**

### Ingredients:

Chickpeas (boiled) – 1 ½ cups

Water – 4 cups

White onion (finely chopped) – 1 large

Diced roasted tomatoes (no-salt-added) – 1 can (15 ounce)

Tomato paste – 2 tablespoons

Garlic (finely chopped) – 4 cloves

Bay leaf – 1

Ground cumin – 4 teaspoons

Paprika – 4 teaspoons

Cayenne pepper – ¼ teaspoon

Pepper (freshly ground) – ¼ teaspoon

Chicken thighs (bone-in and skinned) – 2 pounds

Artichoke hearts (quartered) – 1 can (14 ounces)

Oil-cured olives (halved and pitted) – ¼ cup

Salt – ½ teaspoon

Fresh cilantro – ¼ cup

**Nutrition Information:**

Fat – 15.3 g

Protein – 33.6 g

Carbohydrates – 43 g

**Directions:**

1. Take a large stockpot and add in the chickpeas, tomatoes, onions, garlic, tomato paste, bay leaf, paprika, cumin, ground pepper, and cayenne pepper. Mix well to combine and place it on a medium-high flame.

2. Add in the chicken and cover the pot with a lid; cook for about an hour, stirring occasionally.

3. Once done, reduce the flame to low and take out the chicken and

bay leaves using a tong. Discard the bay leaves.

4. Place the chicken onto a wooden board and use a fork to shred the chicken. Get rid of the bones.

5. Add the drained artichoke hearts and olives and season generously with salt. Stir well.

6. Now add in the shredded chicken and finish by topping it with parsley.

7. Transfer into a serving bowl and serve right away!

## Watercress, Pear, and Roquefort Salad

**Serving Size: 1**
**Servings per Recipe: 4**
**Calories: 101 calories per serving**
**Total Time: 20 minutes**

**Ingredients:**

Strongly brewed tea – 2 tablespoons

White-wine vinegar – 1 tablespoon

Walnut oil – 1 tablespoon

Shallots (minced) – 1 tablespoon

Dijon mustard – 1 teaspoon

Salt – as per taste

Pepper (freshly ground) – as per taste

Red leaf lettuce (washed, air-dried, and torn) – 3 cups

Watercress leaves (washed and air-dried) – 3 cups

Ripe pear (cored and sliced) – 1

Roquefort cheese (crumbled) – 1 ounce

Toasted walnuts (chopped) – 1 tablespoon

## Nutrition Information:

Fat – 3 g

Protein – 6.8 g

Carbohydrates – 8.2 g

## Directions:

1. Start by taking a large bowl and add in the tea, oil, vinegar, mustard, shallots, pepper, and salt. Whisk well until all ingredients are perfectly combined.

2. Add in the watercress and lettuce; toss well until evenly coated. Divide the salad into 4 bowls and arrange pear slices over the salad.

3. Sprinkle each salad bowl with pepper, walnuts, and cheese.

4. Serve!

## Grilled Corn and Veggie Salad

**Serving Size: 1**
**Servings per Recipe: 6**
**Calories: 82 calories per serving**
**Total Time: 1 hour**

## Ingredients:

Corn on the cob (fresh) – 4 ears

Italian salad dressing (reduced-calorie) – ½ cup

Fresh spinach (shredded) – 2 cups

Red cherry tomatoes (cut in half) – 2 cups

Fresh oregano (snipped) – 2 teaspoons

Parmesan cheese (finely shredded) – 2 tablespoons

Fresh oregano – 1 sprig

**Nutrition Information:**

Fat – 2 g

Protein – 3 g

Carbohydrates – 15 g

**Directions:**

1. Start by removing the husk and silk from the corn. Brush all the corn generously with Italian salad dressing.
2. Prepare the grill and bring it to medium heat. Place the corn directly on the grill and cook for about 20 minutes. Turn every 2-3 minutes to ensure all sides are evenly cooked.
3. Remove the corn from the grill and set aside onto a plate. Once the corn is cool enough to handle, cut the kernels and set aside in a large bowl.
4. Add spinach, 2 teaspoons of oregano, and tomatoes into the bowl with corn kernels.
5. Add the remaining Italian salad dressing into the veggies and toss well to coat.
6. Top the salad with parmesan cheese.
7. Finish by garnishing the salad with a few oregano leaves.

## Arugula and Citrus Pork Salad

**Serving Size: 1**
**Servings per Recipe: 4**
**Calories: 272 calories per serving**
**Total Time: 35 minutes**

**Ingredients:**

Pork tenderloin – 1 pound

Salt – ¼ teaspoon

Black pepper – ¼ teaspoon

Canola oil – 1 tablespoon

Orange peel (finely shredded) – ½ teaspoon

Orange juice – ⅓ cup

Rice vinegar – 1 tablespoon

Soy sauce (reduced-sodium) – 2 teaspoons

Honey – 2 teaspoons

Sesame oil (toasted) – 1 teaspoon

Fresh ginger (grated) – ½ teaspoon

Baby arugula – 6 cups

Canned apricot halves (drain and cut in quarters) – ½ cup

Avocado (peeled, seeded, and chopped) – 1 small

Dried apricots (sliced) – ¼ cup

## Nutrition Information:

Fat – 10.7 g

Protein – 25.8 g

Carbohydrates – 18.9 g

## Directions:

1. Begin by trimming the fat off the pork. Cut the pork into slices measuring ¼-inch each.
2. Season the pork slices with black pepper and salt and make sure all the slices are evenly seasoned.
3. Place a large nonstick skillet on a medium-high flame and pour in the canola oil.
4. Once the oil is hot enough, place the pork slices in the skillet and cook for about a minute and a half. Flip over and cook for another

minute and a half. The meat should be slightly pink in the center. Transfer onto a plate and set aside.

5. Take a glass jar with a lid and add in the orange juice, orange peel, vinegar, honey, soy sauce, ginger, and sesame oil. Cover the jar with a lid and shake until all ingredients are well combined.

6. Place the arugula leaves in a shallow serving platter and place the cooked pork slices, dried apricots, apricot slices, and avocado slices on top.

7. Drizzle the prepared salad dressing on top and serve right away!

## Fresh Avocado and Orange Salad

**Serving Size: 1**
**Servings per Recipe: 4**
**Calories: 228 calories per serving**
**Total Time: 25 minutes**

### Ingredients:

Lime-Cilantro Vinaigrette

Fresh cilantro – 1 cup

Olive oil (extra-virgin) – ½ cup

Lime juice – ¼ cup

Orange juice – ¼ cup

Salt – ½ teaspoon

Pepper (freshly ground) – ½ teaspoon

Garlic (minced) – ¼ teaspoon

### Salad

Orange – 2 large

Mixed salad greens – 8 cups

Avocado (diced) – 1

Red onion (slivered) – ¼ cup

Cilantro-lime vinaigrette – ½ cup

## Nutrition Information:

Fat – 18.9 g

Protein – 3.3 g

Carbohydrates – 14.7 g

## Directions:

1. Start by preparing the vinaigrette. For this, add cilantro, lime juice, oil, orange juice, pepper, garlic, and salt to a blender and blend into a smooth, puree-like consistency.
2. Transfer into a bowl and set aside for later use.
3. Use a sharp knife to cut both ends of the oranges and get rid of the peel and the white pith. Remove the membranes of the orange segments and place them into a bowl.
4. Take a large mixing bowl and add in the greens, onion, avocado, and oranges.
5. Pour ¼ cup of prepared vinaigrette on top of the veggies and toss well.
6. Serve right away!

**Note** – The leftover vinaigrette can be stored in the refrigerator for up to 2 days.

# Anti-Inflammatory Vegetarian Mains Recipes

## Roasted Cauliflower

**Serving Size: 1**
**Servings per Recipe: 5**
**Calories: 124 calories per serving**
**Total Time: 30 minutes**

### Ingredients:

Olive oil (extra-virgin) – 3 tablespoons

Turmeric powder – 1 ½ teaspoons

Cumin powder – ½ teaspoon

Salt – ½ teaspoon

Pepper (freshly ground) – ½ teaspoon

Garlic (minced) – 2 large cloves

Cauliflower florets – 8 cups

Lemon juice – 2 teaspoons

### Nutrition Information:

Fat – 8.9 g

Protein – 3.5 g

Carbohydrates – 9.6 g

### Directions:

1. Begin by preheating the oven by setting the temperature to 425 degrees Fahrenheit.
2. Take a large mixing bowl and add in the turmeric, oil, cumin, garlic, pepper, and salt. Whisk until well combined.
3. Toss in the cauliflower florets and ensure all pieces are evenly

coated.

4. Take a baking sheet and place the tossed cauliflower onto the same. Place the baking sheet into the preheated oven for about 15 minutes.

5. Toss over and bake for another 10 minutes. Once done, transfer into a serving bowl.

6. Finish with a drizzle of lemon juice.

## Crusted Mustard Potatoes

**Serving Size: 1**
**Servings per Recipe: 12**
**Calories: 155 calories per serving**
**Total Time: 1 hour**

**Ingredients:**

Yukon Gold potatoes – 4 pounds

Olive oil – 3 tablespoons

Pepper (freshly ground) – 2 teaspoons

Dry mustard – 2 teaspoons

Salt – ¾ teaspoon

Turmeric powder – ½ teaspoon

Mustard seeds (crushed) – 1 tablespoon

Coriander seeds (crushed) – 1 tablespoon

Fresh Italian parsley (chopped) – ⅓ cup

**Nutrition Information:**

Fat – 4 g

Protein – 3.5 g

Carbohydrates – 27.4 g

**Directions:**

1. Start by preheating the oven by setting the temperature to 450 degrees Fahrenheit.
2. Take a baking dish and grease it generously with nonstick cooking spray. Set aside.
3. Peel the potatoes and cut them into cubes measuring about an inch.
4. In a large bowl, add in the oil, dry mustard, pepper, salt, turmeric, and cubed potatoes. Toss until well combined.
5. Transfer the tossed potatoes onto a baking sheet and spread evenly across the sheet.
6. Place the baking sheet into the preheated oven for around 15 minutes. Toss and bake for another 15 minutes.
7. Take the baking sheet and add in the coriander seeds and mustard seeds; roast for another 15 minutes.
8. Once done, transfer the roasted potatoes into a serving bowl and garnish with finely chopped parsley.
9. Serve right away!

## Saag Paneer

**Serving Size: 1**
**Servings per Recipe: 4**
**Calories: 382 calories per serving**
**Total Time: 25 minutes**

**Ingredients:**

Cottage cheese – 8 ounces, cut into 1/2-inch

cubes Turmeric – ¼ teaspoon

Olive oil (extra-virgin) – 2 tablespoons

Onion (finely chopped) – 1 small

Jalapeño pepper (finely chopped) – 1

Garlic (minced) – 1 clove

Fresh ginger (minced) – 1 tablespoon

Garam masala – 2 teaspoons

Cumin powder – 1 teaspoon

Fresh spinach (thawed and chopped) – 20

ounces Salt – ¾ teaspoon

Plain yogurt (low-fat) – 2 cups

## Nutrition Information:

Fat – 24.3 g

Protein – 24.5 g

Carbohydrates – 18.9 g

## Directions:

1. Start by taking a medium-sized bowl and add in the cottage cheese cubes along with turmeric powder.
2. Place a nonstick pan on a medium flame and pour in about 1 tablespoon of oil.
3. Once the oil is hot enough, add in the seasoned cottage cheese cubes and cook for a couple of minutes. Flip over and cook for another 2-3 minutes. Transfer onto a plate and set aside.
4. Pour in the remaining 1 tablespoon of oil and toss in the jalapeno and onion. Cook for about 8 minutes, stirring continuously.
5. Add the ginger, garlic, cumin, and garam masala to the pan and sauté for about 30 seconds.
6. Add in the spinach and sprinkle with salt. Stir and cook for around 3 minutes. Remove from the flame.
7. Now add in the yogurt and mix well to combine.
8. Toss in the cottage cheese cubes and mix until well coated.

9. Serve with flatbread or rice of your choice.

## Spicy Eggplant Bhartha

**Serving Size: 1**
**Servings per Recipe: 4**
**Calories: 246 calories per serving**
**Total Time: 1 hour 15 minutes**

**Ingredients:**

Eggplants – 2 large

Avocado oil – ¼ cup

Onion (chopped) – 1 large

Garlic (minced) – 3 large cloves

Fresh ginger (minced) – 1 tablespoon

Jalapeño pepper (chopped) – 1

Cumin powder – 1 ½ teaspoons

Salt – ¾ teaspoon

Coriander powder – ½ teaspoon

Turmeric powder – ½ teaspoon

Red pepper (crushed) – ½ teaspoon

Tomatoes (chopped) – 2 medium

Fresh cilantro (chopped) – ⅓ cup

Lemon juice – 1 tablespoon

Garam masala – ½ teaspoon

**Nutrition Information:**

Fat – 15 g

Protein – 4.7 g

Carbohydrates – 28 g

**Directions:**

1. Begin by preheating the oven by setting the temperature to 400 degrees Fahrenheit.
2. Take a baking sheet and line it with aluminum foil.
3. Use a fork to prick the eggplants and then place them onto the lined baking sheet.
4. Place the baking sheet into the oven for at least an hour; flip halfway.
5. Once the eggplants are done roasting, scrape off and discard the skin. Place the skinned roasted eggplants on a chopping board and chop nicely.
6. Take a large nonstick saucepan and place it on a medium flame. Pour in the oil and let it heat through.
7. Add in the onion and sauté for about 6-8 minutes. Now add in the jalapeno pepper, ginger, and garlic; cook for around 2 minutes. Keep stirring to prevent the ingredients from sticking to the bottom.
8. Add in the cumin powder, salt, coriander powder, crushed red pepper, and turmeric powder. Stir well.
9. Toss in the chopped tomatoes and cook for about 5 minutes on a medium-low flame.
10. Add in the eggplant, lemon juice, garam masala, and cilantro. Mix well to combine.
11. Cook for about 3 minutes, stirring occasionally.
12. Serve hot with rice or flatbread.

# Vegan Cauliflower Salad

**Serving Size: 1**

**Servings per Recipe: 4**
**Calories: 114 calories per serving**
**Total Time: 15 minutes**

## Ingredients:

Cauliflower florets (bite-sized) – 3 cups

Vegan mayonnaise – ¼ cup

Lemon juice – 1 teaspoon

Dijon mustard – ½ teaspoon

Hot sauce – ½ teaspoon

Turmeric powder – ¼ teaspoon

Salt – a pinch

Celery (finely diced) – 2 tablespoons

Red onion (finely diced) – 1 tablespoon

Fresh dill (finely chopped) – 1 teaspoon

## Nutrition Information:

Fat – 10.3 g

Protein – 1.7 g

Carbohydrates – 4.8 g

## Directions:

1. Take a large saucepan and fill it with water about a quarter way through.
2. Place a steamer basket inside the pan. Place the cauliflower into the basket and cover the pan. Steam the cauliflower for about 5 minutes.
3. While the cauliflower steams, take a medium-sized bowl and add in the mayonnaise, mustard, lemon juice, hot sauce, salt, and turmeric. Whisk until well combined.

4. Once the cauliflower is done steaming, use a potato masher to coarsely mash the same. Use a fork to stir well.
5. Add in the onion, dill, and celery. Mix well.
6. Serve!

## Mediterranean Fresh Lettuce Wraps

**Serving Size: 1**
**Servings per Recipe: 4**
**Calories: 498 calories per serving**
**Total Time: 10 minutes**

**Ingredients:**

Tahini – ¼ cup

Olive oil (extra-virgin) – ¼ cup

Lemon zest – 1 teaspoon

Lemon juice – ¼ cup

Pure maple syrup – 1 ½ teaspoons

Kosher salt – ¾ teaspoon

Paprika – ½ teaspoon

Chickpeas (rinsed) – 2 cans (15 ounce)

Roasted red peppers (jarred and sliced) – ½ cup

Shallots (thinly sliced) – ½ cup

Bibb lettuce leaves – 12 large

Almonds (toasted and chopped) – ¼ cup

Fresh parsley (chopped) – 2 tablespoons

**Nutrition Information:**

Fat – 28 g

Protein – 15.8 g

Carbohydrates – 43.7 g

**Directions:**

1.  Start by adding tahini, lemon zest, oil, lemon juice, salt, paprika, and maple syrup to a large mixing bowl. Whisk until well combined.

2.  Toss the chickpeas, shallots, and peppers into the prepared dressing and combine well.

3.  Place the lettuce leaves onto a shallow serving platter.

4.  Divide the prepared chickpea mixture equally into 4 lettuce leaves.

5.  Serve right away!

## Kale and Bean Stuffed Sweet Potato

**Serving Size: 1**
**Servings per Recipe: 1**
**Calories: 472 calories per serving**
**Total Time: 20 minutes**

**Ingredients:**

Sweet potato (scrubbed) – 1 large

Kale (chopped) – ¾ cup

Canned black beans (rinsed) – 1 cup

Hummus – ¼ cup

Water – 2 tablespoons

**Nutrition Information:**

Fat – 7 g

Protein – 21.1 g

Carbohydrates – 85.3 g

**Directions:**

1. Begin by pricking the sweet potato on all sides.

2. Place the pricked sweet potato in the microwave for around 10 minutes on the highest setting.

3. In the meantime, place the kale in a colander and wash well. Make sure you get rid of any dirt.

4. Place a medium-sized saucepan on a medium-high flame. Add in the kale and cook until it is wilted.

5. Add in the beans along with a tablespoon of water and cook for another 2 minutes.

6. Take the sweet potato out of the microwave and place it on a serving plate.

7. Split the sweet potato halfway through and top it with bean and kale mixture.

8. In a small bowl, add in the hummus along with a couple of tablespoons of water. Mix well to combine.

9. Top the bean and kale stuffed sweet potato with hummus dressing.

10. Serve right away!

## Potato and Chickpea Curry

**Serving Size: 1**
**Servings per Recipe: 4**
**Calories: 321 calories per serving**
**Total Time: 35 minutes**

**Ingredients:**

Yukon Gold potatoes (peeled) – 1 pound

Grapeseed oil – 3 tablespoons

Onion (diced) – 1 large

Garlic (minced) – 3 cloves

Curry powder – 2 teaspoons

Salt – ¾ teaspoon

Cayenne pepper – ¼ teaspoon

No-salt-added tomatoes (diced) – 1 can (14 ounce)

Water (divided) – ¾ cup

Low-sodium chickpeas (rinsed) – 1 can (15 ounce)

Frozen peas – 1 cup

Garam masala – ½ teaspoon

## Nutrition Information:

Fat – 11.6 g

Protein – 8.9 g

Carbohydrates – 46.5 g

## Directions:

1. Fill a large stockpot quarter-way with water. Place a steamer basket into the stockpot and add potatoes into the same.
2. Cover the stockpot with a lid and steam the potatoes for about 8 minutes.
3. In the meantime, place a large saucepan on a medium-high flame. Pour in the oil and let it heat through.
4. Add in the chopped onion and sauté for about 3-5 minutes or until the onion is slightly browned on the edges.
5. Add in the garlic, cayenne, curry powder, and salt; stir and sauté for about a minute.
6. Toss in the chopped tomatoes and cook for at least 2 minutes. Remove from the flame.
7. Transfer the onion, tomato, and spice mixture into a blender and blend. Add about ½ cup of water and blend again into a smooth, puree-like consistency.
8. Return the puree to the saucepan. Add about ¼ cup of water to the blender and pulse to rinse any sauce residue on the sides. Pour it

into the saucepan.

9. Also add the reserved potatoes, peas, chickpeas, and garam masala to the saucepan; stir well to combine.

10.     Cook the potato and chickpea mixture for about 5 minutes before transferring to a serving bowl.

11.     Serve hot with rice!

# Anti-Inflammatory Fish and Seafood Recipes

## Quick and Easy Shrimp Scampi

**Serving Size: 1**
**Servings per Recipe: 4**
**Calories: 316 calories per serving**
**Total Time: 15 minutes**

### Ingredients:

Olive oil – 2 tablespoons

Large shrimp (peel, devein, and pat dry) – 1 ½ pounds

Salt – ⅛ teaspoon

Pepper – ⅛ teaspoon

3 garlic cloves, minced

Red pepper flakes (crushed) – ⅛ teaspoon

Dry white wine – ½ cup

Unsalted butter – 4 tablespoons

Lemon – 1

Flat-leaf parsley (chopped) – 1 small bunch

### Nutrition Information:

Fat – 20.3 g

Protein – 23.5 g

Carbohydrates – 4 g

### Directions:

1. Begin by zesting the lemon and cut it in half. Further cut one half into wedges and set aside.
2. Place the shrimps onto a plate and season them generously with pepper and salt.

3. Take a large nonstick skillet and place it on a medium-high flame. Pour in the oil and let it heat through.

4. Add the shrimps to the skillet and make sure they do not overlap. Cook the shrimps for 1 minute. Flip over and cook for another 1 minute.

5. Transfer the shrimps onto a plate and set aside.

6. Pour some more oil into the pan and add garlic and pepper flakes. Keep stirring and sauté garlic until it turns golden.

7. Pour in the wine and scrape out any browned bits from the bottom of the pan. Cook until most of the wine evaporates.

8. Whisk in 1 ½ tablespoons of butter at a time and whisk well. Season the prepared sauce with lemon juice from half a lemon and salt.

9. Add in the sautéed shrimps, parsley, and lemon zest; toss well until all shrimps are evenly coated. Cook for about a minute.

10. Transfer onto a shallow serving dish and garnish with lemon wedges.

11. Serve hot!

## Herbed Cod with Capers and Roasted Tomatoes

**Serving Size: 1**
**Servings per Recipe: 4**
**Calories: 157 calories per serving**
**Total Time: 15 minutes**

**Ingredients:**

Fresh cod fillets (skinless) – 4 (4 ounces)

Fresh oregano (snipped) – 2 teaspoons

Fresh thyme (snipped) – 1 teaspoon

Salt – ½ teaspoon

Garlic powder – ¼ teaspoon

Paprika – ¼ teaspoon

Black pepper – ¼ teaspoon

Cooking spray

Cherry tomatoes – 3 cups

Garlic (sliced) – 2 cloves

Olive oil – 1 tablespoon

Ripe olives (pitted and sliced) – 2

tablespoons Capers – 2 teaspoons

Fresh oregano – for garnishing

**Nutrition Information:**

Fat – 4.8 g

Protein – 21.6 g

Carbohydrates – 6.5 g

**Directions:**

1. Start by preheating the oven by setting the temperature to 450 degrees Fahrenheit.
2. Take a small bowl and add in the snipped thyme, oregano, salt, paprika, black pepper, and garlic powder. Mix well.
3. Coat both sides of the fish fillets with prepared oregano mixture.
4. Take a baking sheet and line it with aluminum foil. Grease the aluminum foil with cooking spray.
5. Place the coated fish fillets onto the lined baking sheet. Add garlic slices and tomatoes on the side of the fillets.
6. Take a small bowl and add in the leftover oregano mix and oil to the same. Mix well and pour over the tomatoes and garlic. Toss well to coat.
7. Place the baking dish into the oven and bake for around 10-12

minutes. Add capers and olives to the tomatoes and garlic mixture and mix well.

8. Place one fillet on a serving plate and top it with roasted veggies. Serve the remaining fillets and veggies the same way.

9. Serve right away!

## Red Pepper Flavored Quinoa with Salmon

**Serving Size: 1**
**Servings per Recipe: 4**
**Calories: 481 calories per serving**
**Total Time: 15 minutes**

**Ingredients:**

Olive oil (extra-virgin) – 3 tablespoons

Salmon (skin-on) – 1 ¼ pounds, preferably wild, cut into 4

portions Salt – ½ teaspoon

Pepper (ground) – ½ teaspoon

Red wine vinegar – 2 tablespoons

Garlic (grated) – 1 clove

Quinoa (cooked) – 2 cups

Roasted red bell peppers (rinsed and chopped) – 1 cup

Fresh cilantro (chopped) – ¼ cup

Toasted pistachios (chopped) – ¼ cup

**Nutrition Information:**

Fat – 21 g

Protein – 35.8 g

Carbohydrates – 31 g

## Directions:

1. Start by placing a large cast-iron pan on a medium-high flame. Pour 1 tablespoon of oil into the pan and let it heat through.
2. Place the salmon fillet on a wooden board and cut it into 4 equal portions. Transfer to a shallow dish and sprinkle with about ¼ teaspoon of pepper and salt.
3. Place the salmon into the pan (flesh side facing down) and cook for around 3 minutes. Flip over and cook for another 2 minutes. Transfer onto a plate and set aside.
4. In the meantime, add 2 tablespoons of oil, vinegar, garlic, ¼ teaspoon of pepper, and ¼ teaspoon of salt. Whisk well to combine.
5. Also add in the quinoa, cilantro, pistachios, and roasted red pepper. Mix well.
6. Place ¼ of the prepared quinoa mix on a plate and place a salmon piece on top.
7. Serve right away!

## Mustard Flavored Salmon

**Serving Size: 1**
**Servings per Recipe: 4**
**Calories: 198 calories per serving**
**Total Time: 20 minutes**

**Ingredients:**

Salmon fillets (center-cut) – 1 ¼ pounds

Salt – ¼ teaspoon

Sour cream (reduced-fat) – ¼ cup

Mustard (stone-ground) – 2 tablespoons

Lemon juice – 2 teaspoons

Pepper (freshly ground) – as per taste

Lemon wedges

Nonstick cooking spray

**Nutrition Information:**

Fat – 7.6 g

Protein – 29.2 g

Carbohydrates – 2 g

**Directions:**

1. Begin by preheating the boiler.
2. Take a baking sheet and line it with aluminum foil. Grease it generously with nonstick cooking spray.
3. Place the salmon pieces on the greased baking sheet and generously season the fish with pepper and salt.
4. In a small bowl, add sour cream, lemon juice, and mustard; mix well to combine.
5. Spread the prepared sour cream mixture evenly over all the pieces of salmon. Place the baking sheet into the oven and broil for around 10 minutes.
6. Take the salmon out of the oven and place it on a serving platter. Garnish with lemon wedges.
7. Serve!

## Tilapia Fillets Served with Pecans and Orange

**Serving Size: 1**
**Servings per Recipe: 2**
**Calories: 185 calories per serving**
**Total Time: 20 minutes**

**Ingredients:**

Orange – 1

Tilapia fillets – 10 ounces

Salt – ¼ teaspoon

Pepper (freshly ground) – ¼ teaspoon

Unsalted butter – 2 teaspoons

Shallot (minced) – 1 medium

White-wine vinegar – 2 tablespoons

Pecans (toasted and chopped) – 2 tablespoons

Fresh dill (chopped) – 2 tablespoons

**Nutrition Information:**

Fat – 8.8 g

Protein – 16.2 g

Carbohydrates – 11.2 g

**Directions:**

1. Take a paring knife and skin the fish. Also, remove the pith from the orange. Separate the orange segments and set aside in a bowl.
2. Season both sides of the fillet pieces with pepper and salt.
3. Place a large nonstick saucepan on a medium flame. Grease the pan generously with cooking spray.
4. Once the pan is hot enough, place the fillet pieces onto the same and cook for about 3 minutes; flip over and cook for another 5 minutes. Transfer on an aluminum foil sheet and wrap it nicely to keep warm.
5. Add butter to the same pan and let it melt. Once the butter has melted, add in the shallots and sauté for about 30 seconds.
6. Add in the orange segments and vinegar; cook for around 30 seconds. Remove from the flame.

7. Place one piece of the fish onto a plate and top it with dill and pecans.
8. Serve hot!

## Rosemary and Walnut Crusted Salmon

**Serving Size: 1**
**Servings per Recipe: 4**
**Calories: 222 calories per serving**
**Total Time: 20 minutes**

**Ingredients:**

Dijon mustard – 2 teaspoons

Garlic (minced) – 1 clove

Lemon zest – ¼ teaspoon

Lemon juice – 1 teaspoon

Fresh rosemary (chopped) – 1 teaspoon

Honey – ½ teaspoon

Kosher salt – ½ teaspoon

Red pepper (crushed) – ¼ teaspoon

Panko breadcrumbs – 3 tablespoons

Walnuts (finely chopped) – 3 tablespoons

Olive oil (extra-virgin) – 1 teaspoon

1 (1 pound) skinless salmon fillet, fresh or

frozen Olive oil nonstick cooking spray

Fresh parsley (chopped) – for garnish

Lemon wedges – for garnish

**Nutrition Information:**

Fat – 12 g

Protein – 24 g

Carbohydrates – 4 g

**Directions:**

1. Begin by preheating the oven by setting the temperature to 425 degrees Fahrenheit.
2. Take a large baking sheet with a rim and line it with parchment paper.
3. In a small bowl, add in the garlic, mustard, lemon juice, lemon zest, rosemary, crushed red pepper, honey, and salt. Whisk well to combine.
4. Take another bowl and add in the walnuts and panko along with the oil; mix well.
5. Place the salmon on the lined baking sheet and top each piece with prepared mustard and garlic mixture. Spread evenly to ensure the top is fully coated.
6. Now sprinkle the prepared walnut panko mixture on top and spray with cooking spray.
7. Place the baking sheet into the oven and bake for around 10-12 minutes.
8. Once done, transfer onto a serving platter and garnish with freshly chopped parsley and lemon wedges.
9. Serve!

## Garlic-Flavored Roasted Salmon and Brussels Sprouts

**Serving Size: 1**
**Servings per Recipe: 6**
**Calories: 334 calories per serving**
**Total Time: 45 minutes**

## Ingredients:

- Garlic (divided) – 14 large cloves
- Olive oil (extra-virgin) – ¼ cup
- Fresh oregano (finely chopped) – 2 tablespoons
- Salt – 1 teaspoon
- Pepper (divided)
- Brussels sprouts – 6 cups
- White wine – ¾ cup
- Salmon fillet (wild-caught) – 2 pounds
- Lemon wedges – for garnish

## Nutrition Information:

- Fat – 15.4 g
- Protein – 33.1 g
- Carbohydrates – 10.3 g

## Directions:

1. Begin by trimming and slicing the Brussels sprouts. Set them aside in a bowl.
2. Now skin the salmon fillet and cut it into 6 equal portions.
3. Preheat the oven by setting the temperature to 450 degrees Fahrenheit.
4. In a small bowl, add in the oil, 2 garlic cloves, 1 tablespoon of oregano, ¼ teaspoon of pepper, and ½ teaspoon of salt.
5. Cut the remaining garlic cloves in half and toss them with the Brussels sprouts.
6. Transfer the Brussels sprouts to the roasting pan and drizzle with 3 tablespoons of seasoned oil.
7. Place the baking sheet into the oven and roast for about 15

minutes.

8. Add white wine to the remaining seasoned oil and set aside.

9. Remove the baking sheet and mix the vegetables. Spread them out and top the veggies with the salmon pieces. Drizzle the fish with oil and wine mixture.

10. Sprinkle the fish with the remaining oregano, pepper, and ½ teaspoon of salt.

11. Place the baking sheet into the oven and bake for around 5-10 minutes.

12. Once done, transfer onto a serving platter and garnish with lemon wedges.

13. Serve hot!


## Scallops Served with White Beans

**Serving Size: 1**
**Servings per Recipe: 4**
**Calories: 255 calories per serving**
**Total Time: 25 minutes**

**Ingredients:**

Olive oil (extra-virgin) – 3 teaspoons

Mature spinach – 1 pound, trimmed and thinly sliced

Garlic (minced) – 2 cloves

Capers (chopped) – 1 tablespoon

Pepper (freshly ground) – ½ teaspoon

Cannellini beans (no-salt-added) – 1 can (15 ounce)

Chicken broth (low-sodium) – 1 cup

Dry white wine – ⅓ cup

Butter – 1 tablespoon

Dry sea scallops (muscle removed) – 1

pound Lemon (halved) – 1

Fresh parsley (chopped) – 2 tablespoons

## Nutrition Information:

Fat – 8.3 g

Protein – 21.4 g

Carbohydrates – 21 g

## Directions:

1. Start by placing a large nonstick pan on a medium-high flame. Pour in the oil and let it heat through.
2. Add in the greens and sauté for around 4 minutes or until they wilt. Sprinkle ¼ teaspoon of pepper and mix.
3. Toss in the capers and garlic; keep stirring and cook for 30 seconds.
4. Add broth and beans along with wine and let it simmer. Reduce the flame and cover the pan with a lid. Cook for around 5 minutes.
5. Once done, remove from the flame and add in the butter. Stir well and cover with a lid.
6. In the meantime, place the scallops on a plate and sprinkle with the remaining pepper.
7. Place a large nonstick pan on a medium-high flame and add in the remaining oil.
8. Once the oil is hot, place the seasoned scallops in the pan and cook for 2 minutes; flip over and cook for another 2 minutes. Transfer onto a plate.
9. Place lemon halves into the pan with the cut side facing down and cook for about 2 minutes or until they are nicely charred. Remove

from the flame and cut the lemon halves into wedges.

10.      In a serving platter, place the green at the bottom and carefully place the cooked scallops over the same.

11.      Finish by garnishing with freshly chopped parsley and charred lemons.

# Anti-Inflammatory Poultry Recipes

## Grilled Chicken with Cauliflower Rice

**Serving Size: 1**
**Servings per Recipe: 4**
**Calories: 411 calories per serving**
**Total Time: 30 minutes**

**Ingredients:**

Olive oil (extra-virgin) – 6 tablespoons + 1 teaspoon

Cauliflower rice – 4 cups

Red onion (chopped) – ⅓ cup

Salt – ¾ teaspoon

Fresh dill (chopped) – ½ cup

Chicken breasts (boneless and skinless) – 1 pound

Pepper (freshly ground) – ½ teaspoon

Lemon juice – 3 tablespoons

Dried oregano – 1 teaspoon

Cherry tomatoes (halved) – 1 cup

Cucumber (chopped) – 1 cup

Kalamata olives (chopped) – 2 tablespoons

Feta cheese (crumbled) – 2 tablespoons

Lemon wedges – 4 wedges

**Nutrition Information:**

Fat – 27.5 g

Protein – 29 g

Carbohydrates – 9.5 g

**Directions:**

1. Begin by preheating the grill to medium heat.

2. Place a large nonstick skillet on a medium-high flame. Pour in 2 tablespoons of oil and let it heat through.

3. Add in the onion, cauliflower, and about ¼ teaspoon of salt; cook for around 5 minutes, stirring occasionally.

4. Take the pan off the flame and add in around ¼ cup of chopped dill. Stir well to combine.

5. In the meantime, place the chicken into a shallow dish. Drizzle 1 teaspoon of olive oil and rub it nicely all over the chicken. Season it generously with ¼ teaspoon of pepper and ¼ teaspoon of salt.

6. Place the seasoned chicken over the grill for about 8 minutes; flip over and grill for another 7-8 minutes.

7. Once done, place the grilled chicken onto a chopping board and slice it crosswise.

8. Take a small bowl and add in 4 tablespoons of oil, oregano, remaining salt, remaining pepper, and lemon juice. Mix well to combine.

9. Transfer the cauliflower rice into a serving bowl and top with grilled chicken slices, cucumber, tomatoes, feta, and olives.

10. Sprinkle with freshly chopped dill and drizzle with prepared vinaigrette.

11. Finish by placing the lemon wedges on the side.

## Chicken and Veggies with Lemon Couscous

**Serving Size: 1**
**Servings per Recipe: 4**
**Calories: 528 calories per serving**
**Total Time: 25 minutes**

**Ingredients:**

Pearl couscous (whole-wheat) – 1 cup

Tahini – ¼ cup

Water – ¼ cup

Lemon zest – 2 teaspoons

Lemon juice – 2 tablespoons

Olive oil – 2 tablespoons

Salt – ½ teaspoon

Pepper (freshly ground) – ¼ teaspoon

Red pepper (crushed) – ¼ teaspoon

Garlic (minced) – 1 clove

Mushrooms (sliced) – 2 cups

Red bell pepper (chopped) – ½ medium

Coleslaw mix – 4 cups

Baby spinach – 4 cups

Cooked chicken breast (chopped) – 12 ounces

Toasted almonds (sliced) – ¼ cup

Crumbled feta cheese (reduced-fat) – ¼ cup

Fresh parsley (chopped) – 1 tablespoon

Lemon wedges – 4

## Nutrition Information:

Fat – 23.3 g

Protein – 39.9 g

Carbohydrates – 41.5 g

## Directions:

1. Take a medium-sized saucepan and cook couscous as per package instructions. Use a fork to fluff it up and set aside.
2. In the meantime, add tahini, lemon juice, water, 1 tablespoon of oil, crushed pepper, and salt to a small mixing bowl and mix until well combined. Set aside.
3. In a large nonstick skillet on a medium-high flame, pour 1 tablespoon of oil and let it heat through.
4. Toss in the garlic and cook for about 30 seconds. Now add in the bell peppers and mushrooms; cook for about 3 minutes or until the mushrooms release the liquid.
5. Add in the spinach and coleslaw mix and cook for another 2 minutes.
6. Stir in the couscous, chicken, and tahini sauce; mix well and cook for about 4 minutes.
7. Transfer into a serving bowl and top with feta, lemon zest almonds, and parsley.
8. Finish by garnishing with lemon wedges. Serve!

## Ginger and Mango Barbequed Chicken

**Serving Size: 1**
**Servings per Recipe: 6**
**Calories: 244 calories per serving**
**Total Time: 40 minutes**

**Ingredients:**

Mango (peeled) – 1 medium

Ketchup – ⅓ cup

Cider vinegar – ¼ cup

Brown sugar – 2 tablespoons

Tamari (reduced-sodium) – 1 tablespoon

Fresh ginger (grated) – 1 tablespoon

Chinese five-spice powder – ½ teaspoon

Turmeric powder – ½ teaspoon

Chicken drumsticks – 3 pounds

Honey – 1 tablespoon

Salt – ¼ teaspoon

Scallions (thinly sliced) – for garnish

**Nutrition Information:**

Fat – 6.2 g

Protein – 26.1 g

Carbohydrates – 20.6 g

**Directions:**

1. Begin by preheating the grill to medium-high heat.

2. In a blender, add mango, vinegar, ketchup, brown sugar, ginger, tamari, turmeric, and five-spice. Blend into a smooth, paste-like consistency.

3. Place the chicken in a large mixing bowl and add half of the prepared sauce. Toss until all chicken pieces are evenly coated.

4. Generously coat the grill rack with oil and turn one burner to low heat. Place the coated chicken pieces on the grill rack and cook for around 5 minutes, turning every 2 minutes to ensure all sides are evenly cooked.

5. Move the chicken to the lower side of the heat and cook for another 20 minutes, turning every 5 minutes.

6. Return the chicken to the hotter side of the grill and baste with the reserved sauce. Grill for 5 minutes, basting every 1 minute.

7. Transfer the chicken to a serving platter and top with honey. Finish with a sprinkle of salt.

8. Serve with the reserved sauce and garnish with chopped scallions.

# Massaman Chicken Curry with Turmeric Rice

**Serving Size: 1**
**Servings per Recipe: 4**
**Calories: 599 calories per serving**
**Total Time: 50 minutes**

**Ingredients:**

Canola oil – 2 tablespoons

Garlic (finely chopped) – 3 cloves

Fresh ginger (finely chopped) – 2 tablespoons

Brown basmati rice – 1 ¾ cups

Turmeric powder – 1 ½ teaspoons

Rice milk (unsweetened) – 2 ¼ cups

Water – 1 ¼ cups

Salt – ¼ teaspoon

Chicken thighs (boneless and skinless) – 1 pound

Bell pepper (diced) – 1 medium

Red curry paste – 2 tablespoons

Brown sugar – 1 tablespoon

Broccoli florets – 4 cups

Lime juice – 1 tablespoon

Fresh cilantro (chopped) – 3 tablespoons

**Nutrition Information:**

Fat – 19.5 g

Protein – 29.8 g

Carbohydrates – 79.5 g

## Directions:

1. Start by trimming the chicken breasts and cutting them into bite-sized pieces.
2. Place a medium-sized nonstick saucepan on a medium flame. Add 1 tablespoon of oil and let it heat.
3. Add in 1 tablespoon of ginger and chopped garlic; sauté for about a minute.
4. Add turmeric powder and stir well; immediately add the rice and cook for around 2 minutes. Stir occasionally to prevent the rice from sticking to the bottom of the pan.
5. Now pour 1 cup of rice milk along with water and some salt. Let it come to a boil on a high flame.
6. Once the rice milk begins to boil, reduce the flame and cook for around 35 minutes or until the liquid is completely absorbed.
7. In the meantime, place another skillet on a medium flame. Pour 1 tablespoon of oil and add chicken pieces as the oil becomes hot. Cook the chicken pieces for around 6 minutes or until the chicken begins to brown on the edges.
8. Add curry paste, remaining ginger, and bell pepper. Stir well until the chicken is evenly coated.
9. Now add brown sugar and 1 ¼ cups of rice milk; let it come to a boil on a high flame.
10. Reduce the flame to low and add in the broccoli; cover the pan and cook for about 5 minutes.
11. Pour in the lime juice and stir well.
12. Transfer the curry and cooked turmeric rice to separate serving bowls. Garnish the curry with freshly chopped cilantro.
13. Serve the curry over turmeric brown rice.

# Chicken Tikka Masala

**Serving Size: 1**
**Servings per Recipe: 4**
**Calories: 514 calories per serving**
**Total Time: 30 minutes**

## Ingredients:

Canola oil – 1 ½ tablespoons

Chicken thighs (boneless and skinless) – 1 ½ pounds

Yellow onion (chopped) – 1 ½ cups

Garlic (chopped) – 5 medium cloves

Fresh ginger (grated) – 1 tablespoon

Canned tomato paste (no-salt-added) – 2 tablespoons

Turmeric – 1 ½ teaspoons

Garam masala – 1 ½ teaspoons

Cayenne pepper – ¼ teaspoon

Tomato puree (no-salt-added) – 1 can (15 ounce)

Chicken stock (unsalted) – 1 cup

Heavy cream – ¼ cup

Kosher salt – ¾ teaspoon

Black pepper – ½ teaspoon

Fresh cilantro (chopped) – 2 tablespoons

Long-grain brown rice (cooked) – 2 cups

## Nutrition Information:

Fat – 19 g

Protein – 41 g

Carbohydrates – 45 g

## Directions:

1. Begin by cutting the chicken into pieces measuring about 2 inches each.
2. Place a large, heavy-bottomed pot on a high flame. Pour in the oil and let it heat through.
3. Toss in the chopped chicken and cook for about 6 minutes.
4. Now add in the ginger and garlic; cook for about 2 minutes. Keep stirring to prevent the chicken from sticking to the bottom.
5. Add in the tomato paste, garam masala, cayenne, and turmeric powder; cook for about 2 minutes. Keep stirring.
6. Now stir in the stock, tomato puree, pepper, salt, and cream. Mix well and let it come to a boil.
7. Reduce the flame to low and cook for about 10 minutes or until the sauce is thickened.
8. Add in the chopped cilantro and mix well.
9. Serve over cooked rice.

## Spicy Chicken and Quinoa Bowl

**Serving Size: 1**
**Servings per Recipe: 4**
**Calories: 519 calories per serving**
**Total Time: 30 minutes**

## Ingredients:

Chicken breasts (boneless, skinless, and trimmed) – 1

pound Salt – ¼ teaspoon

Pepper (freshly ground) – ¼ teaspoon

Roasted red peppers – 1 jar (7 ounces)

Slivered almonds – ¼ cup

Olive oil (extra-virgin) – 4 tablespoons

Garlic (crushed) – 1 small clove

Paprika – 1 teaspoon

Cumin powder – ½ teaspoon

Red pepper (crushed) – ¼ teaspoon

Cooked quinoa – 2 cups

Kalamata olives (pitted and chopped) – ¼ cup

Red onion (finely chopped) – ¼ cup

Cucumber (diced) – 1 cup

Feta cheese (crumbled) – ¼ cup

Fresh parsley (finely chopped) – 2 tablespoons

## Nutrition Information:

Fat – 26.9 g

Protein – 34.1 g

Carbohydrates – 31.2 g

## Directions:

1. Place the grill rack in the topmost position in the oven and preheat the broiler to half.
2. Take a baking sheet with aluminum foil and set aside.
3. Place the chicken onto the baking sheet and generously season it with pepper and salt.
4. Place the baking sheet in the oven and broil for about 18 minutes.
5. Once done, transfer the chicken onto the chopping board and cut it into slices.
6. In the meantime, add peppers, garlic, almonds, paprika, 2

tablespoons of oil, crushed red pepper, and cumin to a blender and blend into a smooth, puree-like consistency.

7.  In a medium-sized mixing bowl, add quinoa, 2 tablespoons of olive oil, and red onion; toss well to combine.

8.  To serve, take a bowl and place ¼ of quinoa and top it with ¼ of cucumber, broiled chicken, red pepper sauce, and feta. Repeat the same with the remaining ingredients.

9.  Finish by garnishing with chopped parsley.

## Ground Turkey Bowl

**Serving Size: 1**
**Servings per Recipe: 4**
**Calories: 374 calories per serving**
**Total Time: 35 minutes**

**Ingredients:**

Avocado oil – 4 tablespoons

Yellow onion (finely chopped) – ½ cup

Lean ground turkey – 1 pound

Garlic (minced) – 3 cloves

Fresh ginger (grated) – 1 tablespoon

Turmeric powder – ½ teaspoon

Sea salt – ½ teaspoon

Green onion (chopped) – 4 stalks

Carrots (peeled and chopped) – 2 large

Yellow squash (chopped) – 1 large

Broccoli (chopped) – 1 large

**Nutrition Information:**

Fat – 21 g

Protein – 29 g

Carbohydrates – 12 g

## Directions:

1. To make the turkey –
2. Place a large nonstick pan on a medium-high flame. Pour in the avocado oil and let it heat through.
3. Once the oil is hot, add in the chopped yellow onion and sauté for about 3 minutes; stir occasionally.
4. Toss in the ground turkey and stir for about 3 minutes. The meat should be nicely brown by now.
5. Add in the ginger, garlic, sea salt, turmeric powder, and spring onion and mix well. Cook for another 7 minutes.
6. Now add in the chopped carrots, yellow squash, and broccoli; stir well and cook for about 5 minutes.
7. Transfer into a serving bowl and serve with rice or flatbread.

## Teriyaki Turkey Delight

**Serving Size: 1**
**Servings per Recipe: 4**
**Calories: 383 calories per serving**
**Total Time: 20 minutes**

## Ingredients:

Avocado oil – 2 tablespoons

Red onion (chopped) – ½ large

Carrots (chopped) – 2 large

Radishes (chopped) – 1 bunch

Fresh ginger (grated) – 1 tablespoon

Ground turkey – 1 pound

Teriyaki sauce – ¼ cup

Zucchini squash (chopped) – 2 medium

Baby spinach – 2 cups

Sea salt – ½ teaspoon

Chives (chopped) – 1 bunch

Sesame seeds – 1 tablespoon

**Nutrition Information:**

Fat – 21 g

Protein – 31 g

Carbohydrates – 17 g

**Directions:**

1. Take a large saucepan and place it on a medium flame. Pour in the oil and let it heat through.

2. Add in the chopped red onion and sauté for about 3 minutes. Stir occasionally.

3. Toss in the carrots, ginger, and radishes. Cover the pan with a lid and cook for another 3 minutes.

4. Shift the vegetables to one side of the pan and add in the ground turkey. Cook for about 3 minutes; flip the turkey and cook for another 2 minutes.

5. Mix the ground turkey and veggies and stir in the teriyaki sauce, spinach, sea salt, and chopped zucchini. Cover the pan with a lid and cook for about 5 minutes.

6. Transfer into a serving bowl and garnish with sesame seeds and chopped chives.

7. Serve hot!

# Anti-Inflammatory Side Recipes

## Roasted Broccoli with Potatoes

**Serving Size: 1**
**Servings per Recipe: 4**
**Calories: 199 calories per serving**
**Total Time: 45 minutes**

**Ingredients:**

Baby potatoes (tri-color) – 1 pound

Broccoli – 1 head

Apple cider vinegar – 2 tablespoons

Black pepper (freshly ground) – ⅛

teaspoon Olive oil – 3 tablespoons

Lemon (juiced) – ½

Turmeric powder – ½ teaspoon

Cardamom – ½ teaspoon

Salt – as per taste

**Nutrition Information:**

Fat – 7 g

Protein – 7 g

Carbohydrates – 31 g

**Directions:**

1. Start by preheating the oven by setting the temperature to 400 degrees Fahrenheit.
2. Wash the baby potatoes thoroughly under running water and cut them in half.

3. Also, wash the broccoli head and cut it into large but bite-sized pieces.

4. Take a large mixing bowl and add in the oil, pepper, and apple cider vinegar. Mix well to combine.

5. Add the potatoes and broccoli to the prepared oil and vinegar mix. Toss until the veggies are evenly coated.

6. Take a baking sheet and line it with aluminum foil. Place the coated veggies onto the baking sheet. Sprinkle the veggies with turmeric powder, cardamom, and salt. Toss again.

7. Place the baking sheet in the preheated oven and bake for about 20 minutes. Take the baking sheet out of the oven and toss well.

8. Return the baking sheet to the oven and bake for another 20 minutes.

9. Transfer onto a serving platter and finish with a drizzle of lemon juice.

## Roasted Turmeric Sweet Potatoes

**Serving Size: 1**
**Servings per Recipe: 4**
**Calories: 141 calories per serving**
**Total Time: 50 minutes**

**Ingredients:**

Sweet potatoes (peeled and diced) – 2 large

Olive oil – 2 tablespoons

Garlic (minced) – 2 cloves

Turmeric powder – 2 teaspoons

Ground cardamom – 1 teaspoon

Fresh thyme leaves – 1 tablespoon

**Nutrition Information:**

Fat – 7 g

Protein – 2 g

Carbohydrates – 19 g

**Directions:**

1. Start by preheating the oven by setting the temperature to 400 degrees Fahrenheit.
2. Take a large mixing bowl and add in the sweet potatoes, olive oil, garlic, turmeric powder, and ground cardamom. Toss well until the sweet potatoes are nicely coated.
3. Take a baking sheet and line it with aluminum foil. Transfer the coated sweet potatoes to the lined baking sheet.
4. Place the baking sheet into the preheated oven and bake for about 20 minutes. Flip over and bake for another 20 minutes.
5. Once done, transfer the potatoes to a serving platter. Finish by garnishing with thyme leaves.
6. Serve!

## Grilled Citrus Asparagus

**Serving Size: 1**
**Servings per Recipe: 4**
**Calories: 84 calories per serving**
**Total Time: 15 minutes**

**Ingredients:**

Asparagus – 1 pound

Coconut oil – 1 tablespoon

Lemon (zested and juiced) – 1 medium

Orange (zested and juiced) – 1 medium

Salt – ⅛ teaspoon

Black pepper (freshly ground) – ⅛ teaspoon

**Nutrition Information:**

Fat – 4 g

Protein – 3 g

Carbohydrates – 13 g

**Directions:**

1. Start by rinsing the asparagus thoroughly and snapping off the ends.
2. Take a baking sheet and line it with aluminum foil.
3. Place the asparagus on the baking sheet and brush it with coconut oil.
4. Pour the lemon juice and orange juice over the asparagus stems. Also, sprinkle the zest of both lemon and orange onto the asparagus.
5. Place the baking sheet into the oven and grill for about 10 minutes.
6. Once done, transfer onto a serving platter.
7. Serve as a side!

## Grilled Peppers

**Serving Size: 1**
**Servings per Recipe: 6**
**Calories: 63 calories per serving**
**Total Time: 15 minutes**

**Ingredients:**

Bell peppers (cut in large chunks) – 3 medium

Jalapeno peppers (sliced) – ½ cup

Dried oregano – 1 pinch

Mozzarella cheese (shredded) – 1 cup

**Nutrition Information:**

Fat – 3.2 g

Protein – 5.2 g

Carbohydrates – 3.9 g

**Directions:**

1. Start by preheating the grill to medium-high heat.
2. Once the grill is hot enough, gently oil the grate.
3. Place the bell pepper chunks with the inside facing down the grill. Cook for about 5 minutes or until the peppers are slightly charred.
4. Flip the pepper over and place a slice of jalapeno on each of the chunks. Top with mozzarella cheese and finish with a sprinkle of a pinch of oregano.
5. Grill the peppers for another minute or two or until the cheese has melted.
6. Transfer onto a serving plate and serve while hot!

## Italian-Style Spinach and Mushrooms

**Serving Size: 1**
**Servings per Recipe: 4**
**Calories: 199 calories per serving**
**Total Time: 30 minutes**

**Ingredients:**

Olive oil – 4 tablespoons

Onion (chopped) – 1 small

Garlic (chopped) – 2 cloves

Fresh mushrooms (sliced) – 14 ounces

Fresh spinach (washed and roughly chopped) – 10 ounces

Balsamic vinegar – 2 tablespoons

White wine – ½ cup

Salt – as per taste

Black pepper (freshly ground) – as per taste

Fresh parsley (chopped) – for garnish

**Nutrition Information:**

Fat – 14.2 g

Protein – 5.6 g

Carbohydrates – 10.3 g

**Directions:**

1. Start by placing a large nonstick skillet on a medium-high flame. Pour in the olive oil and let it heat up.
2. Once the oil is hot, add in the onion and sauté for a couple of minutes.
3. Toss in the sliced mushrooms and stir fry for around 4 minutes. The mushrooms should begin to shrink.
4. Toss in the coarsely chopped spinach and stir fry for a couple of minutes or until it is wilted.
5. Pour in the vinegar and cook until it is completely absorbed into the spinach.
6. Now pour in the wine and reduce the flame to low. Let it simmer until the wine is also completely absorbed.
7. Season the spinach with pepper and salt; mix well. Top with freshly chopped parsley.
8. Transfer into a serving bowl and serve hot!

## Coleslaw (Sweet and Sour)

**Serving Size: 1**
**Servings per Recipe: 8**

**Calories: 37 calories per serving**
**Total Time: 5 minutes**
**Ingredients:**

Cabbage (shredded) – 4 cups

Red bell pepper (chopped) – 1 medium

Green onions (thinly sliced) – 1 cup

Corn kernels (cooked) – 1 cup

Rice vinegar – ½ cup

No-calorie sweetener – ⅓ cup

Salt – 1 pinch

Pepper – as per taste

Jalapeno pepper (finely minced) – 1

tablespoon Cilantro (chopped) – ½ cup

**Nutrition Information:**

Fat – 0.3 g

Protein – 1.6 g

Carbohydrates – 8.4 g

**Directions:**

1. Take a large mixing bowl and add in the shredded cabbage, red bell pepper, green onions, corn kernels, jalapeno pepper, and cilantro. Mix well.
2. Also add in the rice vinegar, sweetener, pepper, and salt. Combine well.
3. Serve right away or cool it in the refrigerator.

## Simple Roasted Broccoli

**Serving Size: 1**

**Servings per Recipe: 4**
**Calories: 63 calories per serving**
**Total Time: 30 minutes**

**Ingredients:**

Broccoli – 14 ounces

Olive oil – 1 tablespoon

Salt – as per taste

Black pepper (freshly ground) – as per taste

**Nutrition Information:**

Fat – 3.7 g

Protein – 2.8 g

Carbohydrates – 6.5 g

**Directions:**

1.  Start by preheating the oven by setting the temperature to 400 degrees Fahrenheit.
2.  Cut the broccoli head into small florets. Peel the stalk of the broccoli and cut it into ¼-inch pieces. Transfer them into a large bowl.
3.  Drizzle the broccoli with olive oil and season it generously with pepper and salt.
4.  Transfer the seasoned broccoli onto the baking sheet and place the same into the preheated oven for about 18 minutes. The broccoli should be slightly browned and tender.
5.  Transfer to a serving platter and serve!

# Garlic Kale

**Serving Size: 1**

**Servings per Recipe: 4**
**Calories: 87 calories per serving**
**Total Time: 25 minutes**

## Ingredients:

Kale – 1 bunch

Olive oil – 1 tablespoon

Garlic (minced) – 1 teaspoon

## Nutrition Information:

Fat – 4.2 g

Protein – 3.7 g

Carbohydrates – 11.4 g

## Directions:

1. Take a large bowl filled with water and place kale leaves into the same. Soak them for about 2 minutes until you get rid of all the dirt.

2. Remove the kale leaves from the water and get rid of the stems. Coarsely chop the kale leaves and set aside.

3. Take a large nonstick pan and place it on a medium flame. Pour in the oil and let it heat.

4. Once the oil is hot, add in the garlic and sauté for about a minute.

5. Add in the chopped kale leaves and cover with a lid. Cook for about 7 minutes or until it is tender and bright green.

6. Transfer to a serving bowl and serve!

# Conclusion

Autoimmune gear developed by the human body to fight certain diseases, infections, and injuries leads to inflammation. We all undergo inflammation at some point in time. While most of the inflammation gets cured in a short span, certain cases require an expert opinion and an expert diet. This book is all about the latter.

A godsend to those suffering from inflammation, this diet book is a one -stop-shop for answers to almost all queries. For the remainder of concerns, a doctor is always a call away.

One of the most common, beneficial, and highly regarded methods to fight inflammation is to add food items with anti-inflammatory benefits to your diet. Research has shown that anti-inflammatory diet food is much more effective than medicines. When combined with a healthy lifestyle involving regular exercise, an anti-inflammatory diet has proven to be a boon not only for people from regular walks of life but also for athletes in whom wear and tear of muscles and body cells is a common phenomenon.

This book takes care of all the special needs surrounding inflammation, in ways that no one else has been able to achieve so far. This self-explanatory anti-inflammatory diet book not only illustrates tasty recipes but also helps you understand the disease at the core. This prepares you to better fight the cause behind the concern. With so much information available online and offline, it becomes very easy for the reader to get confused and lose interest. This adds to the pain that inflammation has caused already. With the help of this book all, you have to worry about is to stop worrying about anything. Beat the pain while you relish these foods.